Small Meals, Big Joy

The diet that worked to lose weight and other good habits that saved my life

By Sabah Chammas, MD, MAS

This is a self-help book with tools for weight loss and a lifestyle change.

Edited by Danielle Chammas, MD

Introduction

At the age of 72 years (Fahrenheit) and after a lifelong struggle with being overweight, I finally discovered a path that actually helped me lose weight and turn my life around. When I was younger, I was mostly motivated by a desire to look good. There were phases where my weight dropped, but this was never sustained. After growing older and facing my own medical conditions for the first time, I started to seriously consider the health effects of being overweight.

For many years I had tried numerous diets which did not work. I started to look into my eating habits and began searching for an effective diet, but one that was still enjoyable and well-suited to continue as a lifestyle change. My goal was to be healthy especially after I had to have a knee replacement and after developing GERD and some heart issues as well.

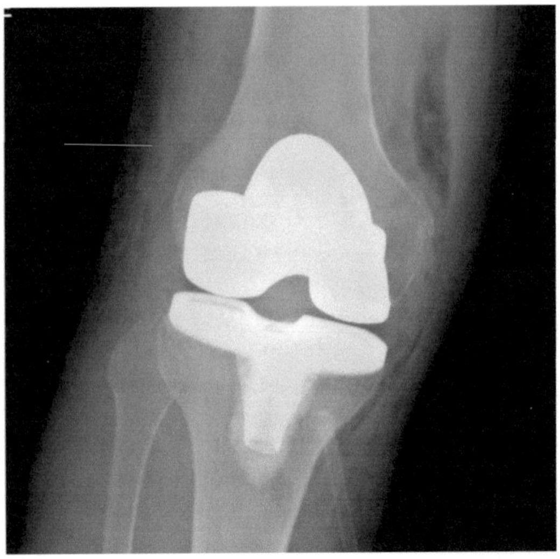

In this book, the path to dietary health that succeeded for me will be laid out. The tools I utilized to achieve more than 45 pounds of weight loss and sustain it will be reviewed. Barriers to success will be explored.

There is no doubt that excessive weight is a complex issue with genetic and metabolic factors at its core. Still, there is a behavioral and addictive component which, if managed well, can help overcome these factors. Alcoholism and drug addiction, for example, have a strong genetic component, yet they can be managed by spiritual and behavioral fitness.

The dilemma is that in all addictions, the universal wisdom is that one has to quit and abstain completely. This of course cannot be done with food. The solution is to identify and avoid addicting foods as well as addictive behaviors and change those. The goal is to have eating habits that are driven by the basic instinct of hunger and not the cravings of addicting foods. This book will show how I did this.

My being a medical doctor who is trained in psychiatry has been helpful. All my medical and mental health knowledge helped me develop the tools of success in order to achieve a sustainable lifestyle change that is based on knowledge and improved spirituality skills like mindfulness. Mindfulness simply stated is to live in the moment and be aware of yourself in that moment in a non-judgmental manner. That means to be present in the moment when you are eating or when you exercise. It means to focus on the food, on your own sensations and on the act of eating. It means being immersed in walking or other exercises at the moment that we are engaged in them. It would be great to have mindfulness in all aspects of life. The best example of mindfulness in my life is when I listen to music. I become taken by the music and the emotions that are triggered by the music. Another example is when I watch movies and become oblivious to all other things.

The book seeks to share the method that was successful for me. It is not meant as a substitute to medical treatment or other dietary guidance, but rather as an additional tool to achieve good health and a successful life-style change. Also, the foods that were chosen seem balanced and contain a variety of nutritional assets, but you need to explore what is essential for you individually. You need to make sure that you are getting enough protein, vitamins and the like. You also need to make sure that you discuss this with your doctor and your dietician.

The book will start with the actual diet that saved my life. The foods, the amounts, the frequency of meals and the actual process of eating will all be discussed. Later on, exercise, psychological factors and barriers to success will be reviewed and many useful tidbits and nuggets will be shared.

Chapter One, The Dietary Plan

The first guiding principle is to eat small portions several times a day. The amount has to be enough to give some satisfaction and some relief of hunger. Planning on eating 6 times a day is ideal. This, in my opinion, is the crucial part of the dietary plan. Different types of lean meats were used such as ground turkey (most often), fish and chicken. Shrimp was included at times. Beef and pork were only consumed on occasion, but this need not be the rule if the portion is reasonable, the cut is lean and if you have a taste for these meats.

Small portions worked so well for me. Not only did I lose weight, but there was no longer this sense of being full or bloated after every meal. Going for walks became so much easier after a meal.

Presence of a healthy amount of bran in the diet is also crucial to success. Furthermore, eating small meals more frequently prevents severe hunger which drives craving and triggers fast eating and addictive behavior in my opinion.

The key is to recognize foods that are addictive and cause cravings instead of normal hunger. Examples would be breaded fried foods with heavy salt and fat content and desserts which are full of sugar and fat. These addictive foods need to be eliminated. A reasonable amount of salt if any was added to the food in my journey to health. After years of addiction to salt, I decided that it is not worth the effect on blood pressure with fluid retention and the like. The same applies to added sugar. Fast food companies have discovered that the combinations of fat plus salt as well as fat plus sugar are both highly addictive and cause cravings. Please consider this and see if it applies to you. Furthermore, minimizing salt and sugar took away a significant portion of the addictive craving part of eating.

No added sugar and no super sweet desserts. That is the only clear-cut restriction in this diet. Don't worry, raisin bran bread is almost a dessert and it is quite healthy. It is almost a bran cake, but it is more like bread as it has no added sugar. You need to prepare it yourself and this way minimize the amount of fat and sugar. The recipe I use for the Bran Bread is listed below with the other foods and it does not have "cups of sugar" or "sticks of butter" like the ones you find online.

In other words, don't deprive yourself. Instead, slowly eat enjoyable tasty things in small portions many times a day and you will lose weight. Combine this with reasonable and enjoyable physical activity and you are well on your way to healthy living. I was actually quite surprised as to how well this worked for me.

Let us take nuts for example. Are unsalted peanuts ok? Many will tell you they are healthy. I avoided them. Why? Because I was not able to control the amount I ate and therefore they are addictive for me. If you can have ten peanuts a day and enjoy them and you are able to stop at this modest amount, then by all means yes you can eat them. If you are like me, then you have to abstain. Once you understand the principle of addictive foods, then you can manage and shape the plan yourself.

Examples of the foods that I used:

1) Meat component: Ground turkey is the staple of my diet, but you can choose fish or chicken instead. Best is to have variety and select a different one each day. Lean Turkey (93% fat free) is ideal because it is nutritious and it is lean with a nice flavor. Adding parsley and some chopped onions to little burger patties and frying it with oil spray in a good pan result in a delicious taste. The patties were somewhat thin and were 2-3 inch wide circles. I had 2-3 of them in one meal with salad.

2) Salad: There are so many choices for good salads and dressings. Lettuce, arugula, spinach, mixed greens etc. depending on your taste. Two of the daily meals had meat with some salad. For a dressing, you can use a touch or flavoring of olive oil, then add Red Wine Vinegar which I love. You can also use other types of vinegar or squeeze a lemon instead. Both go well with olive oil. Be mindful of the quantity of oil, remember a small amount will give plenty of flavor. I avoided all low-calorie products as they tasted like plastic. Remember that enjoyment of the meals is crucial. Allow me also to introduce Taboule' which is a delicious Middle Eastern salad. The basic formula is chopped parsley with chopped tomatoes mixed with cracked wheat. The dressing for this is lemon with a dash of olive oil. I skipped the cracked wheat component in order to save on calories without

sacrificing taste. It still tastes great without it. I personally enjoy eating it alone by scooping bites manually with lettuce. Taboule' without cracked wheat is the epidemy of a healthy food that tastes great. Shredded cabbage with lemon and a dash of olive oil tastes great as well.

3) Bran Bread: This is a huge part of the diet. It has bran which is a very healthy ingredient across different domains. It can lower lipids and turn bowel movements into musical velvet. This is kind of a dessert, but please note that I call this Bran Bread and not Bran Muffins. The difference? Muffins have too much sugar and too much butter. Here is how you make it:
   Dry ingredients: Wheat Bran (2 1/2 cups) with whole wheat flour (1/2 cup only), a little baking powder (2 teaspoons) and baking soda (1 teaspoon). Add some crushed walnuts and raisins, then mix.
   Wet ingredients: Three free range eggs, half a cup of Labne' (Kfir cheese) diluted and whipped in ½ a cup of water, a cup of cranberry or prune juice and two tablespoons of Avocado oil or any vegetable oil. Olive oil flavor does not match well in my experience. Mix them all together preferably manually.
   Now add the dry ingredients gradually to the wet and mix slowly and with kindness. Some people like to use a mixer, but manual mixing is preferred as it promotes mindfulness and a spiritual connection to the ambrosia. My grandmother used to mix food by hand and she was a true food whisperer. This can be had in small portions in between meals, but it is best suited for breakfast. Bake at 350° for around 45 minutes.

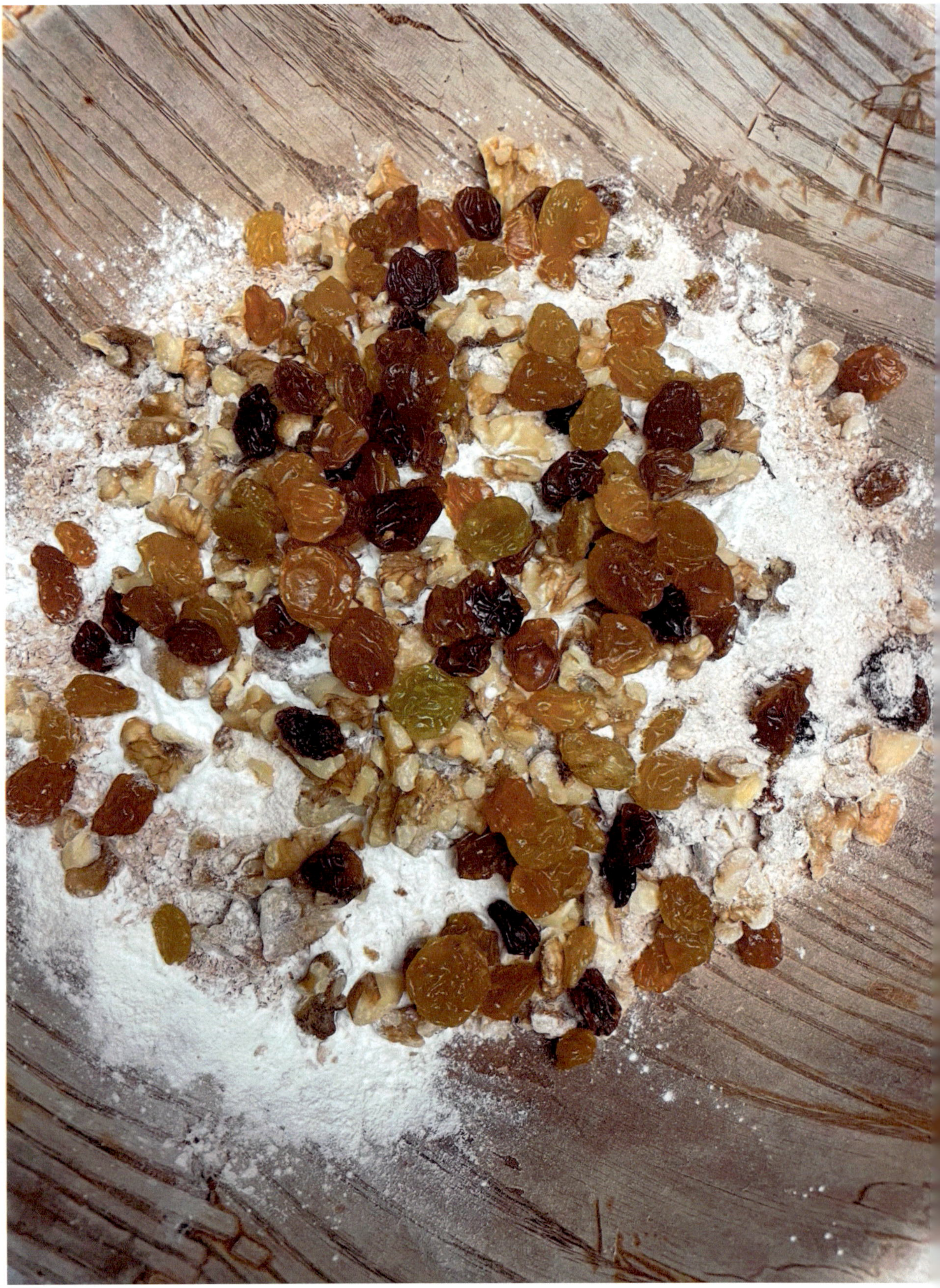

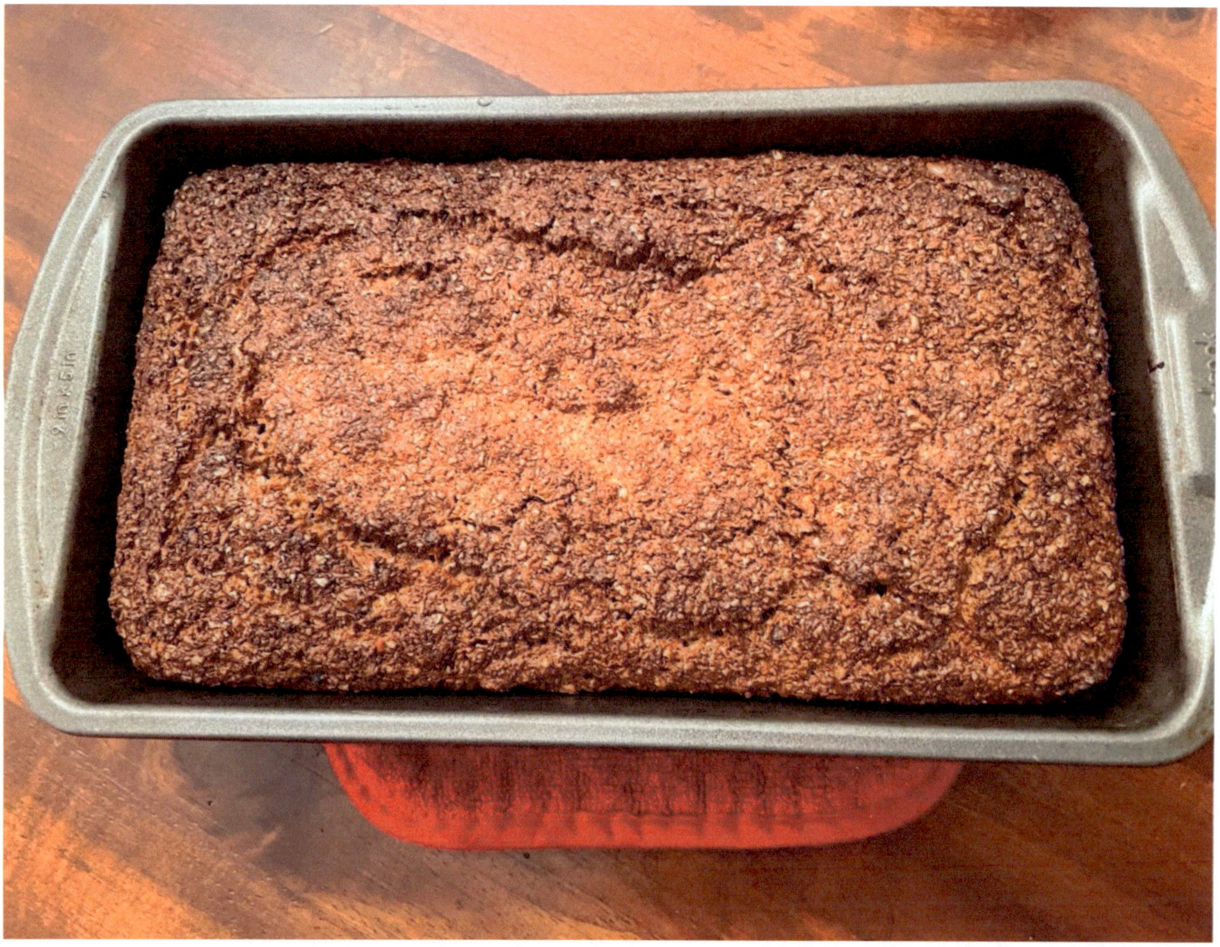

4) Cheese and Labne' (also known as kfir cheese): The preferred cheese is Mozzarella which is low in salt. This can be had with thin sourdough rye wafers which are not as high in calories and carbohydrates as regular bread. The limit is 1-2 crackers per meal. Same can be done with Labne' which is delicious and healthy. Again, remember small amounts. Regular bread was avoided as it would make weight loss much less likely. It's high carbohydrate and calorie content violates the moderation principle of this life style change.

5) Fruits: As a principle, anything that grows from the ground is healthy, but again in modest amounts. Some fruits are healthier than others. Strawberries have the best taste to sugar ratio, that means you get plenty of taste without a lot of sugar. Apples are great and after all, they keep the doctor away provided you have only one a day. Oranges and citrus fruits are rich in potassium and Vitamin C. Some fruits have too much sugar, such

as Pineapple for example. Gain knowledge about the nutritional components and select your food, again in modest amounts.

6) Water and chocolate: yes, please make sure you hydrate well throughout the day. Bran thrives with water. This keeps your vital organs happy and your digestion steady. Dark chocolate 95% to 100% Cacao might taste harsh by itself, but it goes very well with the bran dish. Right hand feeds Bran and left hand feeds chocolate at the same time, ready, GO.

7) Food selections: The foods above are the ones that were included in my diet. You are in no way restricted to these particular items. They are just an example. You are free to change or vary them provided you stay within the same parameters as stated below.

8) Limits (parameters): In summary, it is best to keep your diet with a minimal amount of added salt and with no added sugar. Eat your food in small divided meals. One more important item: try not to mix the different categories above. Meat and salad in one meal. Little snack of bran at a separate time and without mixing other foods. Cheese or Labne' snack by itself as well with thin wafers (thin sourdough rye). A bite of dark chocolate at the end of a meal can serve as a signal to your brain that this meal has ended. Right after that, you can go for a walk. You will be surprised how good it feels to walk after a light meal.

Chapter Two, The Schedule

Described below is a typical day on this diet. All these times are approximate and you manage your schedule as it fits you best:

1) Wake up: Have a slice of Bran Bread. You can have that with sugarless coffee, perhaps with a dash of cream. You can choose on some days to have 2-3 boiled or spray pan scrambled eggs for breakfast, then have your bran later.

2) 10-11 AM: Ground turkey patties with salad and a cracker. On other days you can have chicken or fish.

3) 1-2 PM: Sliced mozzarella or a little Labne (Kfir cheese) with 2-3 crackers or thin wafers.

4) Around 4 PM: Another round of meat with salad or perhaps vary Labne or cheese with sliced tomatoes.

5) Evening: You can have your fruit in the evening. Alternate with a few bites from the bran bread.

6) Additional times: If you have break through hunger in between those times or later, then a small amount of any of the above foods can be consumed. You will become your own master of this good disaster.

In my experience, eating in the evening seems to cause more weight gain, somewhat like the cost of electricity is highest between 4-9 PM.

Chapter Three, The Tools:

Let us start with what not to do. Eating fast and swallowing air not only sounds awful, but it causes problems. One is that by the time you start feeling full, you have already eaten a lot more than needed. That is why you feel full and bloated afterwards. What a terrible feeling. Eating big meals is simply not healthy in so many ways. It is one of the causes of GERD. With small meals, there was no longer a need for GERD medications in my case. The cough that was caused by acid reflux was gone. The weight loss itself helped this tremendously as well.

The trick is to eat slowly. Often, we hear advice to put the fork down between bites. That is good advice, but more important is to savor the food. Chew consciously and appreciate the flavor (mindfulness). Let the taste of the food guide you just like music guides the dancer. Imagine eating less, but enjoying it more. Don't let stress, worry and tension drive your eating. Take a deep breath and simply focus on the here and now. Chew slowly again guided by your awareness. This means you do your best to set aside work and other worries. Nothing exists except your meal in front of you and other good people sitting with you at the table. Be aware of the aroma of the food, the appearance and of course the taste when you chew it

As you grow spiritually, your capacity to do this will strengthen much to your delight. Remember, this skill needs practice and time. Do not expect yourself to be successful on the first day, otherwise you are setting yourself up for failure. You will get better and better at this as you practice it. Each bite becomes a pleasure in itself. A slow pleasure cruise into the taste buds of your mouth instead of a race to satisfy craving.

Eating habits are hard to break. Practice eating slowly and also stopping when your portion is done. Give yourself time to develop this. Hunger will be in much better control with time. Use distraction if you are faced with hunger and craving. What kind of distraction you ask? After your meal, go for a walk for example. This helps with good digestion. It is not only a fun distraction, but also a healthy exercise. Gradually, you will become a joyful walker. Again, give time for this to develop. Good things come with persistence and practice. Remember walking is done for joy even though it is healthy and helpful. It cannot be a chore or homework. The point is to create a new lifestyle based on joyful experiences and awareness of the moment, not one that is driven by craving. A life that is driven by spiritual growth, not one that is driven by guilt. What does the latter statement mean? It means that when you follow simple steps and learn to be aware of your moment, then you will develop a stronger spirit and gain confidence and better control of the mind over the body. In other words, you tame the animal inside you and are able to derive pleasure and enjoyment from food and life in general without the desperate seeking of unhealthy temporary feel-good items. You liberate yourself from the grip of craving for harmful and toxic items and allow your body to be a decent home for your spirit to thrive in.

My awakening began right after my knee replacement in May of 2020 at the height of the pandemic. At that time my weight had gone from the usual unhealthy 259 lbs., which was bad enough, up to 270 lbs. This was alarming and distressing. It was clear that I had no control over the situation. Later on my cardiac echogram and MRI showed that my heart was not pumping very well. They measure ejection fraction (percentage of blood pumped out by your heart muscle after it fills up) which in my case was down to 48% (below normal). Now it is up to 69% without medications as you see in the image below.

Details | Past Results | Graph of Past Results

From: 6/16/16 To: 1/27/22 - or - Latest values: 10

Name *Standard Range*	6/16/16	6/24/21	1/27/22
IVC Diameter *cm*	1.19	2.12	1.61
LA Volume Index *ml/m^2*	23.1	17.8	16.9
LV Ejection Fraction *%*	54	48	69
Mitral Mean Gradient *mmHg*			2.0

Now my weight is 220 lbs. and going down. Hallelujah, a testament to the beneficial effects of healthy eating and of maintaining a moderately active lifestyle. My blood pressure was down and normal. The choice was simple, either surrender and slide down the path to ill health and multiple medications or change my diet and lifestyle all together. An unexpected benefit was a deepening of my enjoyment and appreciation of life.

Here is the report on my cholesterol and lipids, again without medications:

Details | Past Results | Graph of Past Results

From: 1/14/17 To: 2/2/22 - or - Latest values: 10 Apply

View dates as rows

Name *Standard Range*	1/14/17	11/4/17	11/17/18	10/31/19	10/2/20	6/2/21	2/2/22
Cholesterol *<200 mg/dL*	232 H	188	185	233	180	197	164
HDL-Cholesterol *mg/dL*	50	43	43	45	45	46	58
LDL-Chol (Calc) *<160 mg/dL*	170 H	127	127	170 H	116	114	94
Non-HDL Cholesterol *mg/dL*	182	145	142	188	135	151	106
Triglycerides *10 - 170 mg/dL*	62	92	74	89	93	184 H	61

When distraction from cravings is needed, there are many options that may work. Sometimes distraction can be music. If you are feeling down or tense, there is a tendency to munch. Anxiety is often transferred to the jaw and grinding is a known result of it. Give the tension a different path. Listen to music. One of the most amazing effects of music is that it triggers beautiful emotions which can overcome negativity and the clouds that form in our hearts sometimes. The list of potential distractions is endless. Talking to the grandkids over facetime can cure my worst heartache. Don't dwell on the sadness of the past or the peril of the future. Be one with your ground turkey patty instead. Embrace your walk. Dream inside your music. Exist in the moment. Practice this and allow yourself time to develop and to gain strength and confidence. Accept setbacks and take them as a challenge, not as a defeat. In other words, have faith in your ability and do not give up. Weigh yourself once or twice a week. Usually best in the morning before you eat and before you put your clothes on. This gives you a consistent reference point.

Chapter Four, Nuggets and Tidbits

1) Walking is what we humans were designed to do. The basic rule is that it should be fun. If it is enjoyed, then it can be a lifestyle change. That means that walking 5 miles a day is not a realistic life change goal, and it is likely not a lot of fun. Instead, just walk around the neighborhood or in a beautiful park or near the beach. Whatever works provided you enjoy it. Short uphill spurts work for me, but a flat surface walk will do just as well. Keep it under a mile unless the joy of the walk takes you further. Start slow and be patient with your body. If you have a dog, then walking is not a stranger to you.
   Walking is my best friend. It gives me joy in the form of sunshine, sunsets, natural beauty and much more. It helps me when I have negative emotions. It helps me when I need mindfulness. It is a great companion.

2) Water exercises: If you have difficulty walking for whatever reason, then water exercising is an option that is not stressful on the joints. You need access to a body of water of course. Again, follow reason and make sure you enjoy it. Be creative and do any activity that works for you.

3) Weights: During the pandemic, my gym was closed. I improvised a gym at home. Two 5-25 lb. dumbbells did the job. Combine weights with sit-ups and pushups and that is all you need at home. The goal here is not to become Mr. or Mrs. Universe, but simply to stay strong and be in shape. Again, this needs to be fun, although you must admit it is going to be a bit of work as well.

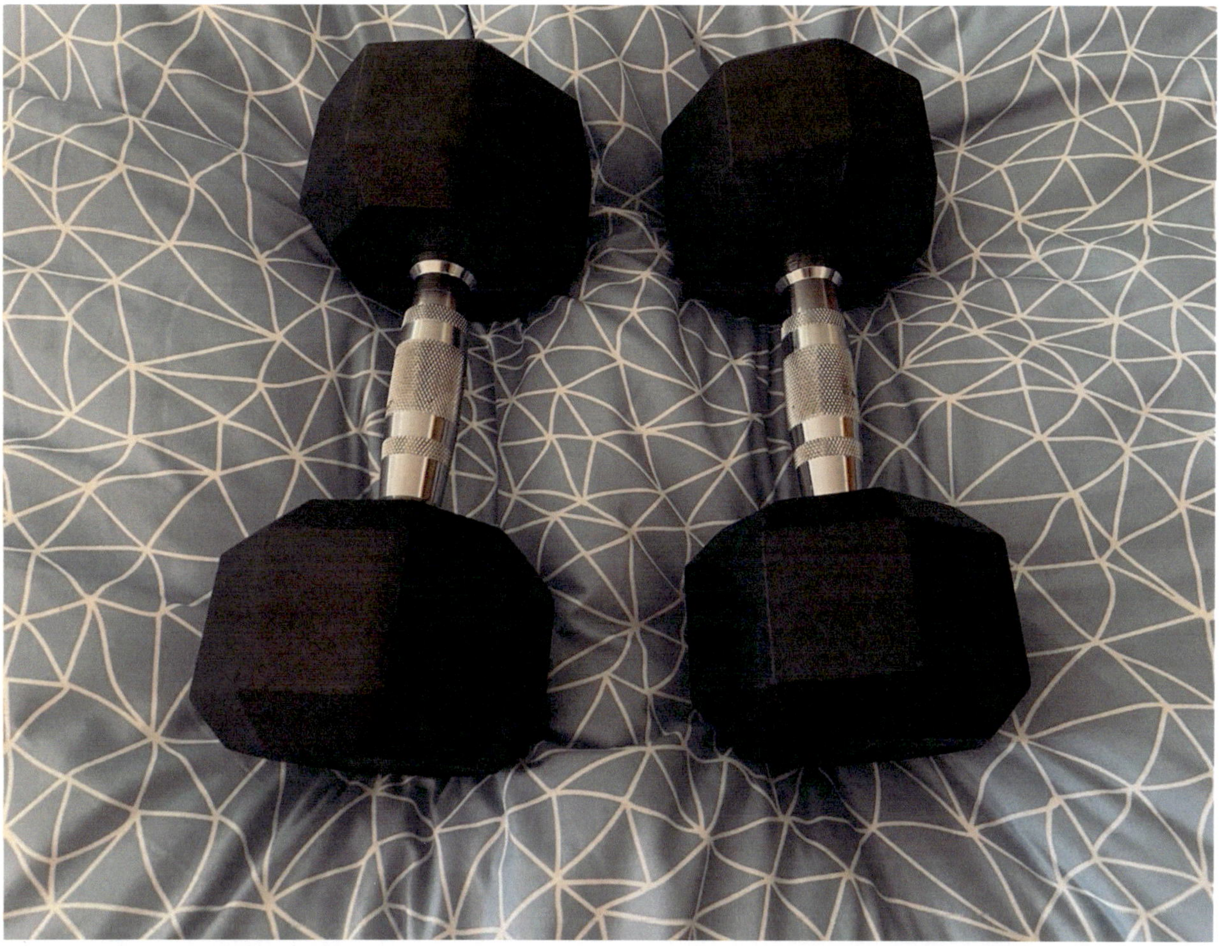

4) Here is my routine: I do 100 isometric sit-ups to start with. I then do straight 12 leg raises while laying on my back with hands below my butt. Then I do the dying cockroach again laying on my back with legs and arms counter flexing about 20 times or more. The dying cockroach is easy and you can increase the count as you please. This was followed by curls (12x2). Then, I do 50 pushups but from the side of the bed while standing as I am older and do not want to stress my musculoskeletal system. You can choose to do push-ups the usual way from the floor. I then finish with modified curls x30. This is a great starting routine which you can build on later if your health allows it of course. In my case, 25 lb. dumbbells are used.

5) Music and dancing: No explanation needed here. I happen to be an avid tango dancer– talk about combining activity with pure joy. Find an activity that you love and do it as often as you can.

6) Medical care: Find a doctor who believes in healthy living and does not jump to medications to solve everything. Luckily, my primary doctor is like this, and she is a great source of encouragement and support. Also, the cardiologist that treated me was willing to wait on medications and give me a chance to do some housekeeping with my body first. It worked. My heart was pumping better, my GERD went away and my new bionic knee is grateful and working very well. All this without medications. Do not get discouraged if you still need medications, it is still a triumph if you have achieved better health.

7) Medical care part 2: Be aware that eating the right way will help many medical conditions, but it is not a substitute for good medical treatment. It simply leads to better outcomes. It is crucial to discuss your diet as well as your treatment with your doctor. This is also not meant to replace or compete with other dietary plans. This book is only meant to provide you with additional tools that will improve your health.

8) Emotional factors: Stress, sadness, fear, anxiety, anger and many other emotions will work against you. We make our worst decisions under duress. Spiritual strength is crucial as in all worthy endeavors in life. Changing one's lifestyle is not easy, but it is doable and it requires time to develop. No matter what, please practice mindfulness. This will insulate you from emotional turmoil. Living in the moment when you are eating helps you set aside emotional factors that may be detrimental to your recovery. Eat slowly, savor your food in every way and enjoy the moment. Your senses and your brain will surprise you if you don't rush them. Much has been written about how mental health has a tremendous influence on eating behavior. If you need more intervention for your mental health, then by all means you should get it. This book only provides tools and information that you can use in parallel to other needed interventions in order to help with dietary and lifestyle change. It is not a substitute for effective evidence-based treatment.

9) Many barriers exist: For example, alcohol contains cheap non nutritious calories. It also stimulates appetite, including the next day. Once your recovery progress and lifestyle changes are established and you have gained strength and confidence, you can resume modest and occasional

social drinking. Buttery popcorn, salted nuts and many other food items need to be avoided. It is my humble opinion that it is easier to simply avoid such foods than to control the amounts.

10) Family: Explain to your family and loved ones what you are doing. Let them borrow this book and read it. They are your allies and they care about you. They cannot help you if they do not understand what you are doing and what is the path you have chosen.

11) Munchies: There are many food items that you can munch and still stay healthy. Oven roasted vegetables of all kinds, such as Broccoli, Cauliflower and even kale leaves can be delicious. You can add pepper or other spices for flavor. I especially like eating lettuce. Be creative and know the foods you are allowing in your body.

12) Television: Arguably the single most weight-adding item ever. Staying home in the evening watching Television is an invitation to addictive eating behavior. It is the same as an alcoholic going to a bar. Try and stay somewhat active in the evening. If you watch a movie, which is one of my favorite things to do, be prepared with non-addictive food.

13) Food availability: Availability of healthy food items that are ready to be consumed is crucial, particularly when you are bored or watching television. Also, when you travel, make sure to have access to bran. During a recent trip to New York, I could not find a bran product from any bakery. I finally found bran muffins in one of the street side kiosks. Be smart, be prepared.

14) Many other examples come to mind, but you need to tailor this whole process to yourself. Take into consideration your likes and dislikes and see how you can fit it in with the dietary and lifestyle changes that are described in this book. Wishing health and wellness to all and hoping this book will save more lives than just my own.

Synopsis:

This is a self-help book with tools for weight loss and a lifestyle change. It tells the success story that led me to lose 50 lbs. It also describes the healthy lifestyle changes that were adopted and how this saved me from heart problems, high cholesterol, GERD, knee arthritis and a general lack of fitness. An added bonus to my undertaking the approach laid out in this book has been an unexpected surge in the joy of living.

About the Author:

Sabah Chammas, MD is a medical doctor who is trained in psychiatry. He has had years of special interest in addictive behaviors and healthy aging. In this book, he shares how he used his knowledge and expertise to wage his own struggle against excessive weight which had affected multiple areas of his health and the quality of his life.

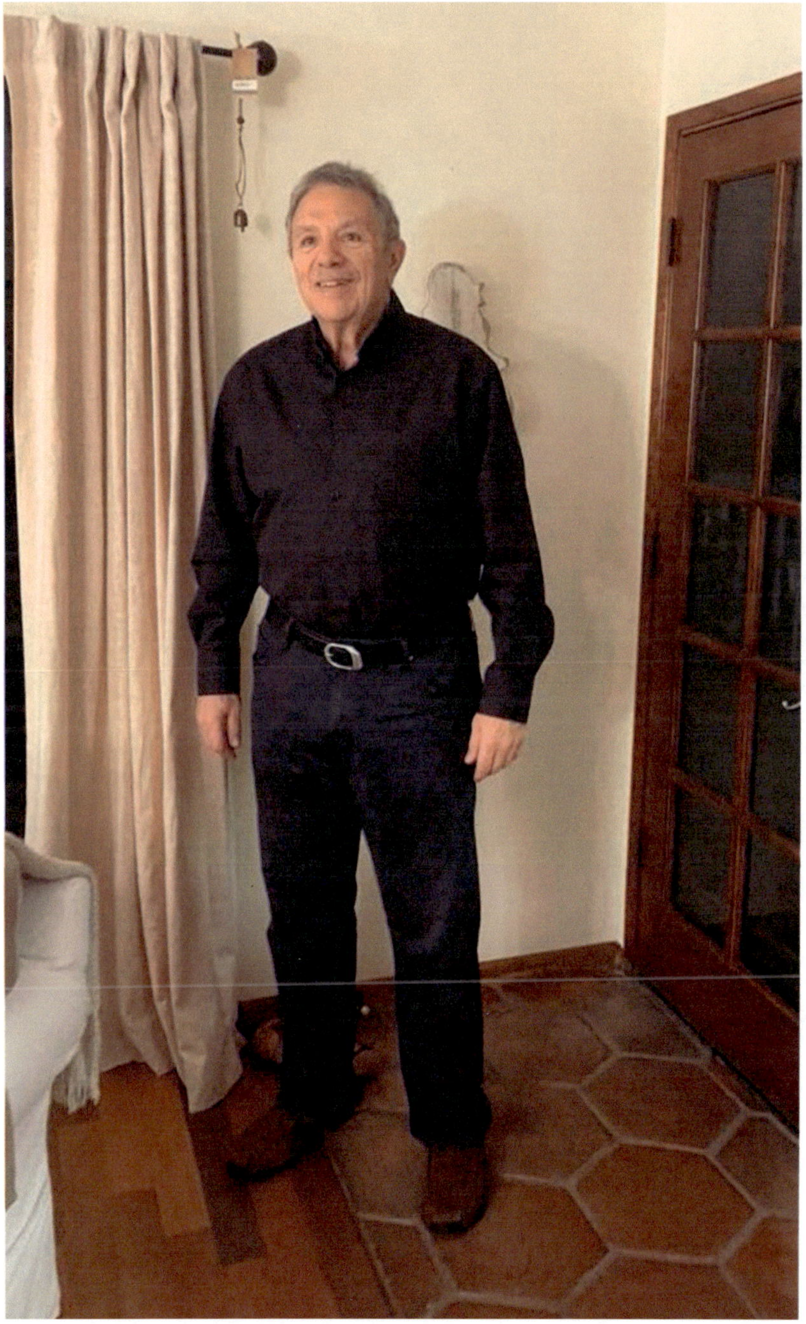

Glossary:

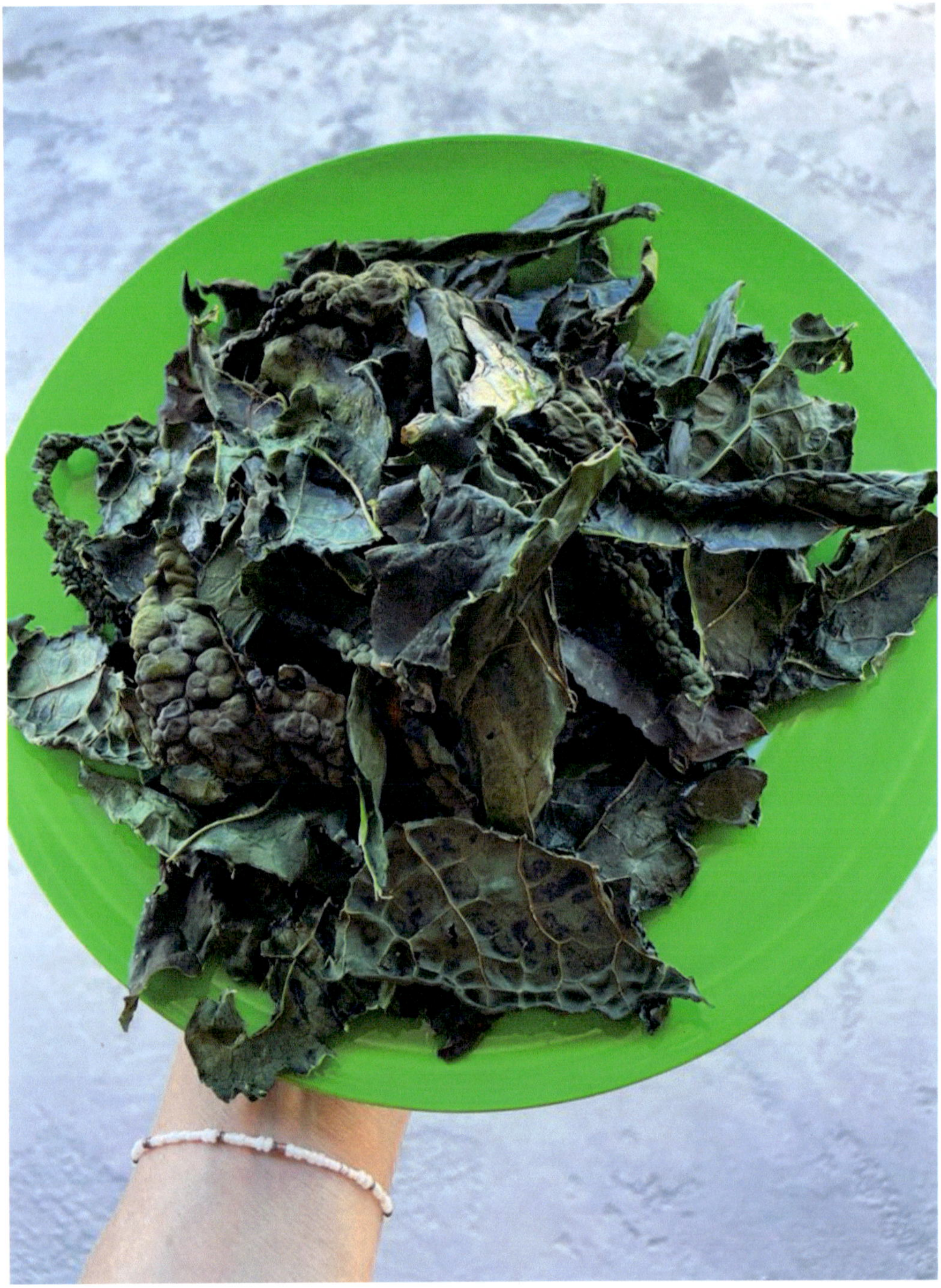

Kale chips roasted in oven.

Bran bread mass production:

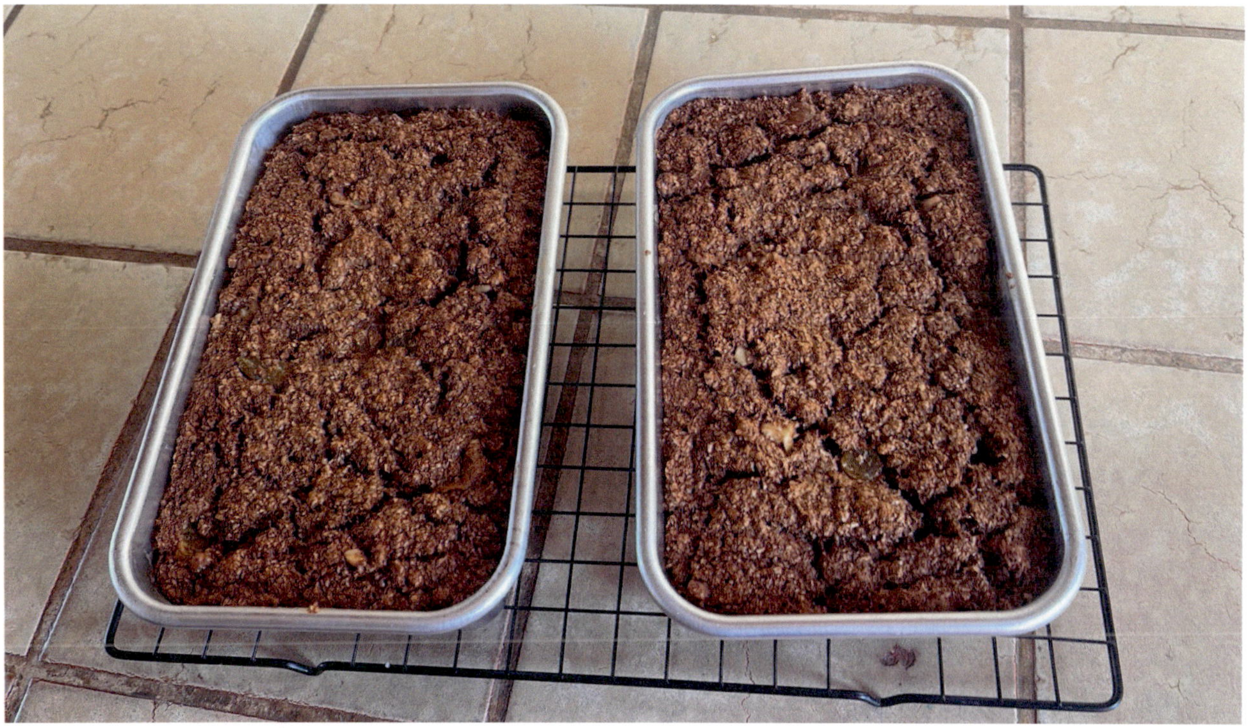

Healthy Mix with Labne:

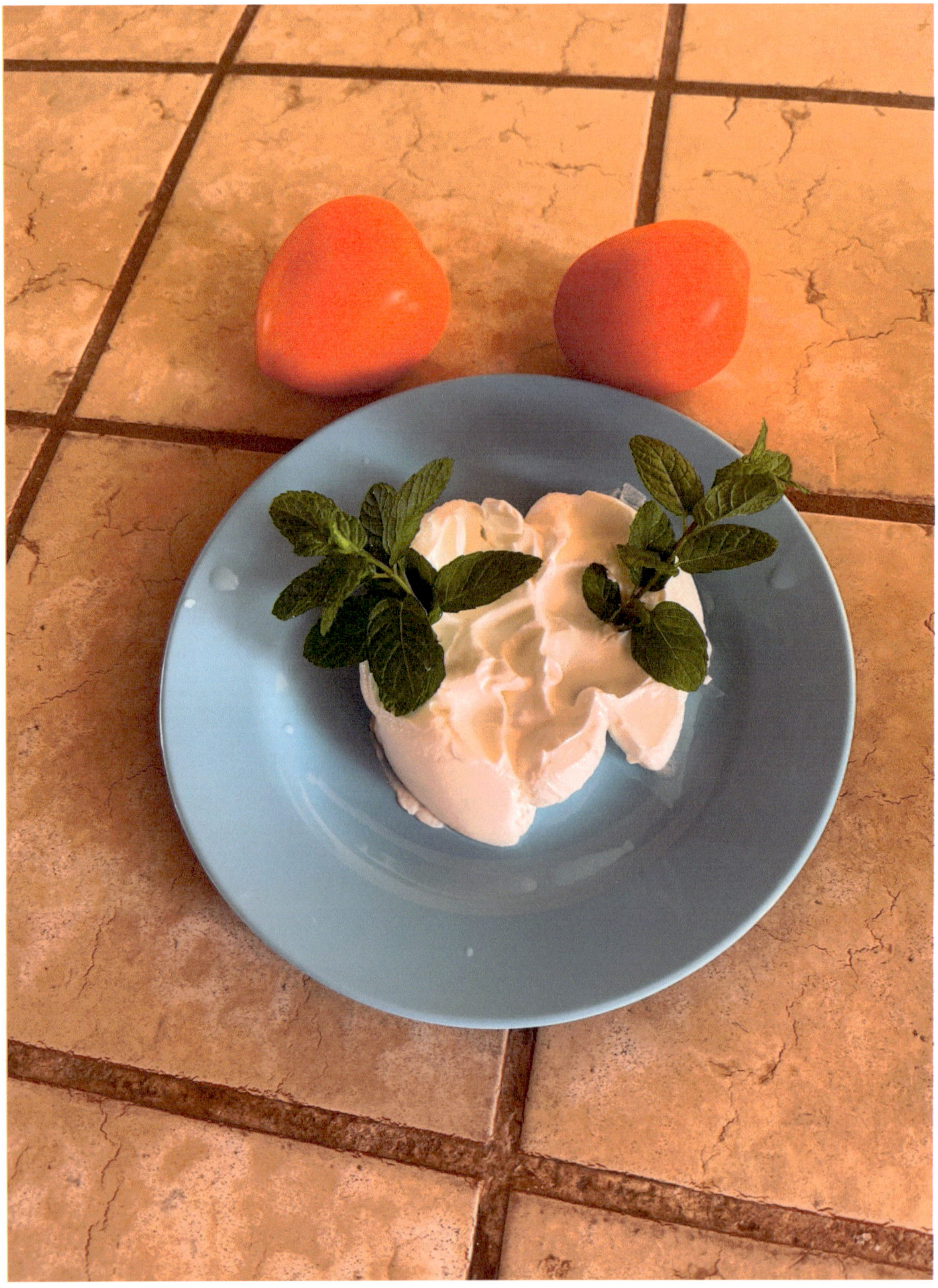

Made in the USA
Monee, IL
05 November 2026

67375732R00017